Emotional Eating

By James Paul

I0428549

Table of Contents

Introduction

Emotional eating is often seen as a taboo topic in the United States, and unless you are suffering from it a stranger to most. Those who face it are certainly not facing a stranger, but rather a deep rooted and severe pain. Emotional eating is a learned coping mechanism thought to alleviate that pain, but if you suffer from the condition you know that is a fallacy.

Inside this book you will find out a great deal of information about the topic to help provide you a better understanding. If you suffer from emotional eating yourself, although I am not a doctor I will help you to find resources to help combat your condition.

We will cover a variety of topics ranging from self checks to see if you are an emotional eater to how you can combat your emotional eating. We will hit on a few myths, and even some truths to the myths. Social acceptance is a massive part of emotional eating at times and that is another topic we will cover.

Not all of the techniques will help you as the human body is not a one size fits all creation. Read this book with a very open mind, and if you are currently seeking help or medical or psychological treatments bring the techniques up. Ask questions!

Here is one of the most important, I feel, points you need to understand. You are not alone, and I pray you realize that yourself. In fact, we will read a few stories of others who have gone through emotional eating and either conquered it or is on the path to doing so.

A Self Test

If you say yes or agree to any of these questions, you may be an emotional eater.

Something inside tells me it is time to eat

When I need to eat, I need to eat NOW

When I'm hungry, it's because of a negative, or positive, emotion

When I eat, I am out there mentally and do not realize what I am doing

I'm full, but I just can't stop eating

I'm hungry, but my stomach isn't rumbling

I ate, and now I feel horrible and the world is going to end

There's something missing in my life and when I think about it I eat

Food protects me from pain

Food will calm me down, for a while, it always does

I see a sign for something, I stop in and buy it

Every weekend we go out and eat at the pizza place until we are going to blow

When I have a headache, I eat

When I'm at a luncheon for work, I'm normally not hungry but don't want to look weird

If the above questions received a yes, you are more than likely an emotional eater. It's not the end of the world though, I promise.

Let's Quickly Dispel a Rumor

We're often told that emotional eating is the same as binge eating. There is actually a clear distinction and difference between the two.

Emotional eating is led by situations, physiological cues, thoughts, society or social settings, and emotions. Binge eating on the other hand is literally eating more than a normal person would eat in a sitting, or day.

To complicate matters even further, binge eating disorder is an extremely serious condition. It is basically regular overeating while the entire time feeling absolutely no control over their eating. Binge eating disorder, based on studies and reasoning, can be seen often as extreme emotional eating. Occasionally many of us overeat, with binge eating disorder it is much more frequently and is typically in binges much like someone with bulimia nervosa. A large difference is that someone suffering with binge eating disorder does not vomit or use a laxative to purge the food from their body.

Eat Your Heart Out: What Emotional Eating Is?

As I mentioned before, emotional eating is the opposite of a victory celebration, it is a painful self inflicted occurrence. Some emotional eaters consume to fill a void or fix a problem. Deep down inside emotional eaters, there is no fixing of any problem. When people, myself formerly (for the most part) included, we create a compounding effect.

The compounding effect I am alluding to is that when we respond to an emotion or emotions by eating, we bring other emotions into the equation. Some of these emotions include a depressed state, guilt, or even temporary complete hatred for ourselves in extreme cases!

Let's understand emotional eating

We know emotional eating is obviously emotionally driven, let's take a look at two examples. One example will be purely an act of gluttony while the other is a sign of emotional eating.

1. After dinner you reward yourself by opening a box and taking a piece of cake and realizing you're not ready to vomit so you grab two more..
2. You look at your phone waiting for a text message, one that hasn't come, and you begin eating a piece of cake. You're not feeling any better, so you eat one more piece, just one more. Before you know it you're exhausted from too many carbohydrates and half of your cake is gone. What isn't gone is that feeling of hopelessness

To those who haven't been diagnosed, or experienced, binge eating the first statement is an obvious choice. In the first statement the individual was eating because they felt like it. The second statement shows the pain that could cause a desire to fill the void opened by sadness with an outside influence. Plainly stated, emotional eating is consuming food, similarly to alcoholism, to fill that emotional need.

Eating once in a while to provide a pick me up or in moderation to celebrate something, a promotion, isn't always bad. If you had a bad day at work and sit down and eat a few pieces of chocolate or a small handful of jelly beans, you're not necessarily using food as a crutch.

Food becomes your crutch when you blow past talking to your significant other and head straight for the fridge. Over time of doing this, you're creating a cycle. Many of the emotions that can contribute to the cycle are:

- Stress
- Mental exhaustion
- Lonely
- Angry
- Upset or sad

There are also two surprising additions to that list to the list above that are obvious emotions. These two emotions are what causes many to become emotional eaters and don't even realize the cycle they are getting into. The two evil additions are boredom and a distracted state of mind. Personally, I found these two to be the most difficult factors to get past when I suffered from emotional eating.

Emotional Eating Sounds Like Addiction

If emotional eating sounds like addiction to you, it should because it can be. The accepted definition of addiction, also bad habit forming, is one that could make you smack your forehead. Addiction is the physiological or psychological dependence, as on a substance. Another definition of addiction is the condition of using something on a regular or dependent basis.

It may seem like something you've heard again, however when we cover coping mechanisms it will make sense, is that emotional eaters are addicted. I've dealt with numerous addicts in my life and although some mental health workers disagree I see emotional eating and alcoholism as very similar. It would be fair to also throw recreational drug use into that realm.

I've found the arguments above emotional eating not being an addiction to be incomplete in their findings. Like addiction, you use the crutch which is food instead of a drug like alcohol to get your "fix". When you're eating, especially in the early stages, you may feel much better however the problem still exists.

Subconsciously this new found addiction is another compounding issue to the condition in that you stop finding healthy ways to deal with emotional distress. The "fix" you sought from eating is very short term, and often times you feel far worse than when you started. This is when other emotions start to creep in.

Just like as with other types of addiction, emotional eating is often caused by triggers, which we covered above. In severe cases, a therapist may need to intervene.

Non Emotional Eating Triggers

If you feel like you understand emotional eating and the triggers, I'm going to throw a wrench into your thought process. Aside from emotional eating led specifically by emotions, there are 4 other triggers that can cause emotional eating. Keep in mind that each of these triggers can be broken down exponentially and this is only to cover the main groups.

Physiological "emotional" eating is caused by a physical sense. Some people will eat because they have a headache, which can sometimes be a sort of hunger pang. One of my issues was skipping meals and randomly being hungry.

Situational is, I feel and have noticed based on society, a large percentage of emotional eating. Think of this as literally nothing more than "when" eating. When sitting down to watch television, a handful of chips can easily turn into an empty bag. It doesn't stop with the sofa and television. When passing a billboard for a new sandwich you may stop in and grab one. Movies and sporting events can contribute to "when" eating also.

Thought based emotional eating may not be the largest, and it is by no mean small, but can be one of the most painful. This, I feel, is the most painful of emotional eating occurrences and as we touched on above is often to fill a void.

Social eating can be triggered often times by a lack of confidence, or esteem issues. When out with a group that orders a pizza for example where each slice is easily 800 or more calories. You know you shouldn't take a slice, however your group is eating rapidly and you long to be one of them.

Although there are four types of emotional eating and all can and should be recognized and addressed, thought based is seen by many to be the worst. If you ask a thought based emotional eater, there is none worse. Aside from techniques to aid in combating emotional eating, the main focal point of this will be the thought based eating.

The Social Stigma

Have you heard the saying "people are mean" recently? You probably have, the United States as a matter of fact seems to be getting more rude and ruthless toward other people by the day. You can blame a lack of censorship, too much television, pop music, or social media. Regardless of how or why, it's a known and painful truth. Looking at the numbers on any knowledgeable source, you will read that the suicide rate is growing, fast. A lot of suicide has to do with an inability to control emotion.

The inability to control emotion doesn't always have to include suicide, but it does often bring with it sheer darkness. We've all been through it at some point, bullying that is. We've all also gone through pain of being picked on. One of the biggest bullies we will face is often on the other side of the mirror looking back at us. Out of the statements below, can you relate to any of them?

"I'm a loser"
"I will never amount to anything"
"I'm a pig"
"I'm a failure"
"Why can't I look like them?"

"I wish I could fit in"
"How did I get so big?"
"I shouldn't be like this, but I have no control*".

Those are a few samples, the list will obviously take up a book in itself. I mentioned at the end of the foreword that you aren't alone, I was with you. I can relate to times where I said those same things. Although you may not be told those directly from another person, and if you have been that is emotional abuse, you say them to yourself.

I had done it for years personally, self down talking which I will discuss in my "story". We as emotional eaters put undue pressure upon ourselves to fit into an accepted mold. It's unfair, again, to blame any form of media as we feed ourselves. At time there seems to be absolutely no hope, but what is feeding us? We are physically doing it ourselves.

*This could be a sign of binge eating disorder

How Can We Stop Emotional Eating?

One common method toward stopping emotional eating is to engage in "groups". The groups I am referring to are in a social setting and not necessarily group therapy. After reading about social eating, you may be very worried about eating in a group setting and rightfully so.

One fix toward preventing social emotional eating could be to set ground rules before you go out. Tell yourself you will not eat an unhealthy choice, you should receive no weird looks when you say you're trying to eat healthier. In fact, that may aid your confidence or esteem slightly when people congratulate you on embarking on bettering your health.

Form the right kind of relationships with the right people. Close family outside of those you deal with regularly work as a wife may share the same habit, addiction, or emotional eating whichever way you chose to label it.

Beg for accountability! I added an exclamation to that statement to evoke emotion and make you want to act. When you write something down it has a great chance of getting done which is common knowledge. However if you ask for people to watch out for you and your eating, they're more prone to act as a support team for you!

Getting physical has shown time and again to help people dramatically reduce the occurrence of emotional eating. As a former certified personal trainer I am very partial to this and have heard numerous, ridiculous in my opinion, recommendations. Some will tell you when you are hungry to go out and take a walk. It sounds great at face value, however if it is January and you live in the northern part of the United States it is not plausible. Here are a few, better, options than simply go for a walk:

- **Do a push up and when you are done do another one.** Here's the caveat, you may be for example 100 pounds overweight and push ups are not only painful impossible, but dangerous as well. I understand however you do not need to perform the push up from a complete plank. You can do push ups on your knees, or on stairs as well. Doing them on stairs may actually be a great place to start as you are using leverage to your advantage.

- **Use a vacuum.** It may sound funny at face value, however this is an exercise that many people I trained started off with. It's actually extremely easy as well. To perform a vacuum you contract your abdominal muscles. After you control them, you hold that contraction and breath in slowly. When you exhale is when you do a vacuum, you begin contracting your abdominal muscles even more. It may sound impossible, but it isn't. It is like a partnered stretch where they push you down more a little bit after you exhale.

- **Do a few types of crunches.** That is not a typo, when you feel like eating or sense your cue, do some crunches. I would start with the traditional crunch and perform a few of those, maybe 5 to start with. Ater 5 of those, immediately do a few reverse crunches. A reverse crunch is where you start with your knees at a 45 degree angle and use your lower abdominal muscles to raise your pelvis (and feet) about 3-6 inches off the floor. After that crunch variety, lay fully extended on the floor, place your arms to form a T shape and lift your feet about 3 inches off the ground. If this is tough for you, hold this position for about 5 seconds and lower them, resting for 5 seconds and repeating. If you are able to do this comfortably, raise your feet and legs about 6-12 inches slowly and lower them.

What I am recommending above has worked for quite a few of my clients. One extremely important things to note is that when performing physical activities is to monitor your pain levels. There is a strong difference between an exercise burn and pain. If you feel pain, stop immediately and consult a doctor which I am not.

You can do the traditional walking, the best way to exercise when you feel you are going to eat emotionally is to have fun. If you are a thought based emotional eater physical activity is going to allow you to feel endorphins which will be released into your bloodstream. Endorphins are basically an emotional internal morphine. How can you have fun? Let's create another short list:

- Have a "potato sack race", with family or friends is better

- Dance
- Play on the ground with a pet or child

The next idea to aid in halting emotional eating is to create a journal. Hear me out on this before you write it off, I journaled the wrong way like you probably have. When journaling you're not just writing down what you ate and what emotion you felt. You need to write down what led up to that as well. The next idea with your journal should provide your "a ha" moment, review it. Focus on writing your details so you have an idea in 3 weeks what you wrote about and why it is on the list. Here could be an example journal:

Monday: I had breakfast and when I saw my child's mother called me I got upset. I sat for about 20 minutes after I saw she called and couldn't get out of my way fast enough to hit the fridge. I grabbed a slice of cheese, a can of coke, and grabbed a few cookies. I had to get my mind off of her and fast so I sat and watched TV. I swore I ate a chip or two, but half the bag I opened yesterday was gone and I really don't remember eating that many. I really felt like crap and ate the rest of the bag.

The story above may seem fictitious however one of the stories you will find shortly in this book is from my friend. That is a literal portion of his journal he allowed me to read with him.

Something else happens, and I alluded to it earlier, when you write something down. It has a better chance of happening. Another component of the benefit to writing isn't just the potential for action but the fact it is gone. You wrote it down and you let it out of you. If you have extreme esteem issues and find it near impossible to talk about your issues, this could work wonders for you.

Finding motivation is another amazing way to help in combating weight loss and work on emotional eating. If you do something for no reason, there is a strong possibility the action will stop and you will move on. When you are motivated to do something however, you are willing to embark and there's a sense of need and obligation to work toward the desired end result.

Something you should do that resembles journaling is to carry a small pocket notepad with you. When you find yourself thinking negatively, stop what you are doing and write it down! Compile a small list and transfer them to your journal. This list is going to help you alter your own train of thought.

A sample note could be what I wrote before.

"I'm a loser"

"I will never amount to anything"

"I'm a pig"

"I'm a failure"

"Why can't I look like them?"

"I wish I could fit in"

"How did I get so big?"

"I shouldn't be like this, but I have no control".

That list is going to need some explanations from me, and your list will need explanations from you as well! Let's go line by line:

"I'm a loser" What makes me a loser? Because I eat and shouldn't? It's an issue I WILL conquer!

"I will never amount to anything" I won't if all I do is comfort myself with food and allow myself to use excuses

"I'm a pig" A pig has 4 legs and hooves, I am a grown man

"I'm a failure" Everyone fails, did I quit or use my motivation to press on?

"Why can't I look like them?" Because I do not have the same genes as them. I am my own unique person.

"I wish I could fit in" Am I stopping myself from fitting in? Because they won't hang out with me, am I using my emotions to prevent others who want to be with me from doing so?

"How did I get so big?" I ate a lot, often times too much. It's cleanup time and I am taking advantage of this new slate.

"I shouldn't be like this, but I have no control". This is my challenge, when I feel I am losing control, I force myself to do the opposite.

The list above is literally something I found handwritten. I always asked my children why they felt a certain way, and when they couldn't come up with an answer, their mood changed. My daughter would quite often say she was mad, I would ask her at what and when she replied she didn't know i reminded her she obviously had nothing to be mad over. Her mood would change rapidly.

One thing you need to do is not allow yourself to search for excuses to feel that way. Reasons are fine however an excuse is just that, an excuse with no basis.

If you notice my list, you will notice it is a list of opposites. The left side is extremely negative, the right side that is not italicized is positive. The positive is the next way to overcome emotional eating which is through the use of affirmative or positive thinking.

Positive thinking is something that most consider to be absolutely foolish or impossible. If you ask a bikini model they may feel that emotional eating is false as well, it's all opinion and experience. The model doesn't show signs of emotional eating while we know there is a deep pain behind it. With emotional eating, the thought based form primarily, there's a very strong chance you let the "negative' rule your thought process.

Positive and negative thought patterns have been studied extensively, and are readily available to research yourself. I won't bore you with case studies, however I can say there is overwhelming evidence that both attitudes and perceptions can cause you to act. In fact it has also shown that psychosomatic symptoms can be seen from emotion or mindset. To prove the idea of positive thinking, let's look at G.I.G.O.

G.I.G.O. is an acronym for "garbage in garbage out' and the thought process behind the topic is extremely easy to understand. If you are feeding your mind negative thoughts, you will be more prone to exert negative emotions. The same with positive thoughts. One way to see how this can work is with a car air filter; pardon me as I am not a mechanic. An air filter traps all sorts of nasty things before it enters the cabin, or where you drive in a car. When the filter is clogged with too much undesirable items, junk for a lack of words, it will begin spitting them out into the air you breath in the car!

Another method toward breaking the habit, or addiction, to emotional eating is to meditate. This is also something I do not want you to write off as not for you. Proper meditation can open your mind, quite easily, to notice and subconsciously prevent yourself from slipping up! More importantly is something I have experienced myself, which is to picture your body the way you want it to be.

I was an extremely heavy, no pun intended, cigarette smoker. I felt the wheeze and cough come on extremely strongly one day when I swore I had pneumonia. I was told it was smoker's cough and I learned a tip from my father. When I couldn't breath, I needed to picture my black lungs as becoming cleaner with each breathe. At first i wrote it off, and eventually mindfully gave it a shot. It worked well as I set a timer for 5 minutes and meditated solely on the thought that my lungs were becoming cleaner!

What worked for me at one of my darkest levels may not be encouraged by a doctor. I got tough on myself, very tough. In our society we are taught and nurtured to baby ourselves. Looking back generationally we can see a softening of the American character and demeanor. Being a slight history buff I will concur it is due to the fact we need to simply "feel". The issue with this comes from the fact that if we get too accustomed to simply making ourselves feel good, no matter the situation, we risk avoiding reality. Taking one of my notes I had written down and shared before, can be a great way to illustrate this concept.

"I'm a failure", that is something many of us will say to ourselves. At face value it is extremely harsh and blunt, and it also offers no course to rectify the attitude. When I added *"Everyone fails, did I quit or use my motivation to press on?"* I did not try to emotionally coddle myself. I accepted reality and forced myself to answer my own question. In fact at many times I did use it as an excuse. It was difficult to admit to myself, however if you cannot be honest with yourself, you're going to continually slip up.

Going along with being harder, or more blunt with ourselves is treating ourselves more like children. Children are forced into receiving will power, however as adults we train ourselves to feel like "I deserve it". It is similar with cigarettes as well as with emotional eating and even a gambling addiction.

If a child was upset and wanted a snack, and you know about the problems with emotional eating, would you let them have it? It's not just any snack, it's a quarter pound cup cake. You would surely make them wait a while, and more than likely cut it up yourself correct? Treat yourself like a child, it's very rational however you picked up the habit many of us face with instant gratification. It's not easy to teach an old dog new tricks, and if you've developed a habit of craving here are a few tips that should work extremely well for you in cutting back your emotional eating.

Don't fear the fridge, but make it accountable. For many of us, the refrigerator is where a lot of our weaknesses lay. Picking your vice shouldn't be tough chocolate sauce, coffee creamers, cheese, pies, and others. If you want to add the freezer to this we can add microwaveable "appetizers", ice cream and other frozen desserts for example. You obviously can't get rid of your refrigerator, but you can do a few things. Put a lock on your fridge and put a sign in and out sheet on the key, strategically located at the other end of your house. What the signing in and out process will do is show you how often you are actually using the refrigerator.

Create rations. This tip is somewhat time consuming, but very easy. Take a plastic bag and purchase a kitchen scale for your snacks. Although this works excellent with any food, we'll assume you're not cooking a few steaks when you're upset. Place one half of the available size in the bag, and write on it that the bag contains one serving.

Watch your time. I have heard of the rumor that you need to eat every 2 hours, which is what led to a lot of my success. The fact of the matter is that if you have a desk job and 3 hour daily commute, you're sitting for roughly 11 hours per day. If you're not physically active due to lifestyle demands such as dropping your children at events then eating every 2 hours is somewhat foolish. What you can do is plan your main meals roughly 4.5 hours apart, and plan for a small snack every 1.5 hours. If you're like the majority of American's you have a smartphone with an alarm clock. Set alarms to go out through the day for each meal and snack. If you're a habitual "I'm bored" eater, sticking to this tip should cut back your emotional eating tremendously.

Pass on your chores. Doing this as a child was probably a pipedream, however it could be a real possibility as an adult. I have gone on planned food shopping trips with clients in the past and noticed something very interesting. If they were left to a list, they would still end up with a cart that is 15-20% more than what they had planned if there was no meal plan in place. With a meal plan, their shopping trips would end up much better, however they were still straying from their list. When they had their meals planned and a shopping list focused solely around their meal plans, with a few healthy snacks, the shopping trip ended with only the list being purchased. The caveat was this occurrence in my experience was far more difficult. If you're week when it comes to temptation, swap lists with a family member or friend. Give them the money and your list, and do the same for them.

Aim high, but realize nobody is perfect. Defeat is difficult for anyone, however it is a part of life. If you try the tips above and do alright, but mess up a few days due to a sheer emotional catastrophe, fix yourself and start over. Tell yourself time and again that mistakes happen, but give yourself the respect of vowing to try harder! When you wake up if you ate a little more than you should have at night you have a fresh start in the morning. If you ate 3 bags of rations at 10 AM, stick to the plan the rest of the day.

Write yourself notes. Earlier you learned about the benefits of positive thinking. I have used these same notes myself, along with keeping my letter handy and can attest toward them working. At the end of this book I will give you a few notes to write and stick around your house.

You deserve a reward. When you are doing a great job tracking what you do, watching your notes, locking the refrigerator and hiding the key, reward yourself. One thing I had noticed quite a bit when it came to people failing while I was training them was they didn't allow a cheat. Cheating is illegal on your taxes, and is asking for failure when quitting smoking, however cheating on a diet is acceptable. I in fact encouraged clients to use their cheat as an attainable goal. If you have left the ice cream sandwiches alone in the freezer and fought temptation, eat one at the end of the week. Write a note and stick it on your freezer that you earned your cheat and be proud of your accomplishment. I wouldn't recommend increasing the goal more than you originally set it.

Using these tips should help you quite a bit, I hope you put them into action!

Real Emotional Eating Success

If you feel that emotional eating is going to be the end of your life and there is no turning back, the stories will show that is not the case. Many feel failure, myself included. i will begin with my journey, and tell you ahead of time there were a few slip ups. There was also a variety of triggers, some of which occurred at the same time.

To provide agreed upon anonymity, the last name and pictures of the individuals will be left out. Their area will be stated and everyone is from the United States. Each individual was interviewed with interview style questions, and their stories are true however edited to fit into a story type of form.

I hope you find encouragement from these stories, and maybe try the tips the way others have. After my own story I will be giving the story also of some of my personal training clients, including a few who had tough and remarkable journeys.

My Story

Growing up I was more than fit i was actually underweight for most of my life. I was a Boy Scout and Royal Ranger, a similar but Church based program, and was active in a variety of sports. I played baseball, soccer, wrestling, and touch football. I was more than fit, I was an athlete in the making.

My first experience with emotional eating was during the end of a rough spell at high school. I was still running a lot, however it was during a troubled time where we were fighting or running from the police. I would regularly smoke marijuana with "friends", and that led to starvation as I was only 15 and had no job for money. When i got home, i would normally splurge on things my parents had laying around. I can tell you my mom had the best snack food and leftovers ever, but then again everything tastes great when you're under the influence.

This trend carried on for over a decade. When I was officially kicked out of high school, I didn't have to go to bed at 9:00 and wake up at 6:00 for school, so my eating would eventually start at work when I made munchie food, and carry on to 3 in the morning when I would make more food. Eventually I picked up drinking as well, adding my caloric value. I also became trained to where I was a complete situational eater and would only eat when I was under the influence.

I didn't balloon at this point yet, however I went from 150 pounds to 200. I looked fit still, however my 6 pack was gone. I would go out to dinner and have no desire to eat anything, unless I had a beer. I would actually enter the restaurant seemingly aggravated, and I was. As soon as I had a shot, I was a new person and had no problem shoving my hand toward the appetizers.

If we stopped at McDonalds, I would order 2 Big Mac meals and a milk shake. If I was with a group, i would keep ordering food and eating until the rest of the group was done. This was a bad move because I was always known to devour food, hardly chewing it.

When I was 20, I was arrested twice in a year and chose to serve a jail bid and plead to charges instead of face 18 months for violating probation. I kicked myself for taking the bid as I was innocent, however I was going to be going to jail regardless. If you think school lunches were rough on the palate, you have no idea what jail food is like. When I got out, we went to celebrate, with a curfew and permission from my parole officer. I remember taking a bite of loaded mashed potatoes and falling in love with food. I came out of jail around an acceptable 160 pounds and was quickly back to 200.

Being without my friend and no access to marijuana or alcohol, I followed the rules, I quickly turned to food. The things I saw, coupled with a loss I had been suffering from emotionally since I was 8 made me feel something was needed. Something to take my head off of things, I couldn't speak with any of my friends either so in a way I was completely alone.

The more I ate and slept or watched television, the more I hated myself. I would walk by the refrigerator and eat something just to eat something. My ex girlfriend was with me through the ordeal and actually encouraged me to get some help. By the time I was 22 years old, my stomach went past, but not over, my pants for the first time. I felt massive failure and extreme hatred for myself.

I continued eating and saw my body change in a bad way, I also saw my optimistic attitude change even more dramatically. I knew I was eating far too much but had no idea why. It didn't click until I saw first hand that I had no control. My ex girlfriend's 8 year old nephew wanted to challenge me to a few pushups. At the end of the competition he did 2 pushups and I couldn't lift myself off the floor.

Parole had been over for a little while now, and there was no restriction on alcohol or marijuana any longer. I began using them again, and fell back into my situational eating. Instead of starting slowly I would eat as I had previously, however this time I was also eating lunch and dinner and consuming I would say 4-5,000 calories a day. I was over 300 pounds now and emotionally I was falling flat on my face. It came to the point that I would no longer remove my shirt during intercourse, and eventually any time I had to walk by a mirror. To this day i am almost never fully naked aside from going into a shower.

To say emotional eating is horrible is an understatement, it is complete and utter Hell. I was a very heavy personal trainer, my clients loved my knowledge base however I always saw them looking at me. They looked at me with, in my own mind, "why don't you take your own advice" written over their face.

A true desire to change really came when I was roughly 26 years old. I was sober when another ex girlfriend pointed out the fact i could open a bottle of gin around noon and polish it off before 8 PM. I was smoking marijuana like it was cigarettes, and smoking almost a pack and a half of Newport 100's per day. I realized I had a problem, when my son told me I looked like Santa Clause without the beard I knew I was going to change.

The Change, And the Hiccups

I knew I was going to change, and like i told my clients to write a letter stating their motivation and what led them to where they got, I wrote my own. The contents will not be disclosed, but I will say I read it quite a few times during the first few months. If you're expecting me to say that change is easy, it's not. However, the challenge is worth more than undertaking and I cannot begin to list the beneficial experience I had as a result.

If I didn't see a picture of me standing in my Royal Ranger uniform, I can't say I would be writing this book as a "work in progress" success story. I saw my physique, and I looked good. But what hit me more was the memories I had of when i could literally pray all of my problems away. I missed that feeling, and started to pray again. I prayed all throughout my incarcerations, but never found the faith and love I had for my God as when i was a youth. Before I lost my weight, there were things I had to work on.

I began really writing a lot of lists, such as the one I wrote before. I also wrote down what I knew to be my triggers. I was very aware of the point I was a burnout and was going to forget so I put a piece of paper near the refrigerator, couch, arm chair, and microwave. If I was eating it, then I was going to write it down first and why i wanted it. I didn't stop myself, I wanted to know what I was eating, but more importantly why. I forced myself to do this, and it was a pain. I noticed I didn't write half the things down, because I was high. I got so mad at myself, I sat and ate. I wrote down why I was eating a plate of buffalo tenders, because I was a failure.

Honesty is the BEST policy

When I wrote down I was a failure I realized two things, one was that I couldn't do this alone. I found myself praying to God that He PROMISED me that I could do all things through Christ who strengthens me. The second thing that hit me was that I should have written down my feelings for myself a while back.

I was always confrontational, it went hand in hand with fighting during my earlier years. I loved a fight and I loved to compete. I hated to lose and I remember staring in the mirror and shouting loud enough to wake someone who was in my house. It was a "friend" and she asked what was happening. I told her it was time for me to put up or shut up, and while I was still buzzing from my gin and grapefruit juice I dumped the rest of the bottle on the front lawn while I smoked a cigarette. My dead friends needed it more than me. God doesn't help those who refuse to help themselves. I was going to change.

The lists were still all over the place and I remember it being a Sunday, I smoked a joint and headed toward a list. I wrote down that I didn't work hard enough to satisfy my munchies. I also knew if I didn't eat they would soon be gone, not soon but within an hour or two. I remember before I went to bed that I wrote down that I won that night. It was something that remained in my wallet until I had lost that wallet.

I fulfilled the munchies with a better option, and although they didn't go away, I knew they wouldn't stay. I had a Muscle Milk shake and sipped it slowly, not inhaling it as I normally do. I also did about 30 minutes worth of isometric exercise which helped keep my mind off of eating. I won't lie, I was starving, but the hunger went away when I began meditating on "I can do all thing through Christ who strengthens me".

I didn't quit smoking, although I was surely done drinking, and I got the munchies regularly. I remembered telling quite a few clients about being an 'evil ruler' to themselves. Not letting themselves enjoy something, especially when they stay on track. I also knew I didn't particularly enjoy dropping $18 on 6 packs of protein shakes. I began rationing my food a little bit, specifically for the midnight munchies. I would put a few appetizers on a plate and set them aside in the refrigerator or freezer. After about 4 months of this, my ex (who I was extremely unfaithful to) decided to leave. I was glad as she was a nice girl, but I was with her for the children. I also lost my job at Vitamin World after being set up by who I thought was a best friend. The job bothered me far more than losing her as I was done with her emotionally for a while at that point.

When I had nothing aside from my children on the weekends, I sat back one day before going out job hunting and looked at my records. I peaked at 335, and wrote down that in a year I would look less like Santa Claus. About 4 months later, not exactly to the day, I saw something. When I was "failing" and finally gave Christ "the wheel", I still failed, however the win rate gave me a 89% winning record. What is more staggering is I had been getting wins on a much more, almost weeks straight, basis for the last 2 months. I was winning even though I didn't accept that until I sat and looked at my progress. I was also down to 298! To me that was huge, and I was wearing XL shirts instead of XXL or even 3XL!

I failed a few times after that, and I saw at time week long set backs. I have always had high expectations for myself based on my accomplishments as a child. One thing I did notice is I was far more accepting of the idea that I could start a new slate whenever I wanted and try harder. At the time of this writing, I am under 230 pounds. I still smoke, however that is going to be my next victory.

Sammi's Story

Sammi grew up in rural Virginia, where a tradition was home cooking. Her mother was a vegetarian and used a lot of soy based meats. Sammi grew up very active and around horses, a fit young girl. As her grandmother and grandfather began watching her more often as she aged, she found she liked their food, "real food" much tastier.

Through the years, Sammi would eat with her mother when she was hungry as she was developing a taste for sweets and meats. She was steadily putting on weight. At her grandparents house she wouldn't eat when she was hungry, she would eat all day long. She would often times eat to the point of nausea.

In junior high school, she was placed on a strict diet for her weight through the help of a nutritionist. She managed to lose some of her weight, and ate more healthily. When she entered high school, she took a baking class and found her love of sweets again.

"I would eat healthy for a few years after I lost most of the weight I put on. When I joined my baking class though, I realized I was eating whenever I did homework, which was baking and cooking. I never liked school, but I had no problem doing my 'homework' for the baking class. I was great at it, placing in numerous competitions."

Sammi went back to her diet, however found when she was doing homework she would eat. She started thinking about what she was doing to stop her eating, and decided she was no longer going to be doing her homework in the kitchen. She would also make sure to have a small, healthy, snack before she started doing her home work.

"When I set the rule of eating before my homework instead of while I was doing homework, I saw I was losing about 1-2 pounds per week. I started riding horses more and contracted my ab muscles and used good posture for exercise. I was actually doing great for a while and got a job working at a college cafe. I didn't necessarily gain weight while working there, but I did afterwards in a big way."

When Sammi began working, she enlisted the help of a personal trainer. Aside from working out he put her on a diet. It was far off of what the nutritionist had her doing, he wanted her to consume 2,600 calories daily.

"I got into the habit of eating 5 or 6 times each day, 5 on a normal day and 6 when I worked out. I wasn't losing or gaining any weight, and then I lost my job."

When Sammi lost her job, she found she was still eating but only when she would look at the clock. "I became depressed, I wasn't working and had a newborn and when he would sleep it was around when I use to eat. So I would sit on the couch and eat."

Sammi continued the pattern of situational, and emotional, eating. She ballooned to almost 280 pounds and she had it.

"I was always large chested, however I looked at the scale one day and saw my stomach was past my breasts, I couldn't see my feet. I knew I needed changes and I did. I would take James' tips and apply all of them. I was screwing myself, James recommended that I try no more than a few tips at a time and get use to forming habits. I'm not a model, however I have lost a good deal of weight."

For the record, Sammi is gorgeous and also is now my wife. That is probably one of the best perks I have found of being a personal trainer. Sammi went through a number of situational eating "relapses".

"The biggest tip I can give anyone when it comes to beating back the urge to eat when you're not hungry is to be mindful. It's not easy, a few times I would catch myself eating over emotions and think 'I'm already eating, who cares'. Eventually, I would take a lot of thought into the idea that I DO have that clean slate."

Beatrice's Story

"I grew up in a very close knit Portuguese family. We lived upstairs above my grandmother and I would visit her all the time, she was my best friend. I grew up loving food, however was active with sports all year long. If you know anything about the Portuguese people, you know we can cook. I learned from my grandmother and often times everyone told me that they couldn't tell if I made the meal or her."

As the years grew on, Beatrice's grandmother aged and she helped her cook regularly. Upon the passing of her grandfather, Beatrice would work and quickly became her grandmother's caregiver. Beatrice came home from work and went to give her grandmother her medicine. She opened the door and assumed her grandmother had fallen asleep, she was not responding to Beatrice. As Beatrice opened her grandmother's bedroom door, she saw she was in bed with what Beatrice described as "a warm, beautiful smile."

"I walked in and saw her hand stretched out as if she was holding my grandfather's hand. I really think he was sent to guide her home. I kissed her cheek and she was so cold, I knew she was gone. I remember my world crashing. I was depressed for weeks, and when I thought it was getting better I would look at my drive way and just break down and cry.

I began cooking food and imagining my grandmother. Although it was only me at the house, my family had grown and moved away, I was cooking large meals to feed many of us. It was my way of staying with my grandmother. I would eat the food all day, often finishing half of a meal set up for 8 people."

Beatrice fell into the emotional eating trap that many find themselves in. She would have thoughts of her grandmother which would result in acting as a trigger, making her want to eat to get past her loss.

"I was fat, and there was nothing I could do about not eating. I wasn't so much as happy when I ate, but it felt like the only way I could share time with my grandmother. I knew I needed to change my habits as my doctor told me I was on the verge of diabetes and had high blood pressure and cholesterol."

Beatrice tried dieting, only to find that she became more depressed and would overeat as a result of her "failings". "I ate all day everyday at one point, getting up to over 350 pounds. I couldn't even walk up stairs. I knew I couldn't eat as much as I was, but I did anyway. I felt like food owned me."

Beatrice went to the hospital on numerous occasions with chest pain, fearing it was a heart attack. One day I was talking to a therapist a work colleague told me about and she opened my eyes. She only had to ask me why I don't carry a photo of my grandmother with me. I started to do that, and i even wrote down things my grandmother would say or do. Memories. I found that overtime I didn't eat quite as much but I still had a long way to go. What helped me was a group of people I work with went walking, and I asked if I could go with them. I told them what I was doing, and my friend Cynthia would call me a few times a night to check on how I was doing. I had good days and bad days, but when I put the effort in it was a lot easier than I thought."

When suffering a loss, it's often difficult to "plug the void" and makes food the easiest culprit. I asked Beatrice how she managed to stay on track as at my gym she was upset often. "My grandmother didn't want me to be hurt ever, and when I want to cook and eat to feel I am with her I could see her in my head shaking her finger at me. I know she did not go in pain, and I started to think she was a lucky one, a lot of people have to hurt when they go. She lost her weight and she is in Heaven with my grandfather, they are together again. I have my life and always smile at her picture now and remember her beauty and don't cry when I see her."

John's Story

John regularly denied being an emotional eater, in fact he would often times swear he had a complete grip on his eating. He could never answer the question of how he got so large however, and at times toyed with the idea of a stomach reduction surgery. He came to me puzzled one day at the gym and asked me if I had any ideas because the screening deemed him ineligible. I had him write down what and when he ate.

What made me curious if John should see a doctor was that he ate very regularly, meaning at the right times. He ate the right foods as well. I did see a few days each week where he managed to forget to write anything in. He compiled a new list and put it on his refrigerator as I recommended he do. The information didn't change I asked him how much he ate and that is when things began to click.

"Honestly, i felt a lot of shame on some days when I would eat. I broke down in James' office because he couldn't help me if he didn't know what was going on. It made perfect sense, but it hurt so bad. I didn't skip eating on some days like the one's I left blank but I would almost literally clean out my pantry.

When I was growing up, I would get sad like any other kid. I would always get something to eat because my parents told me it would make me happy and I guess in a way it did. Over the last 5 years I would get sad almost all the time. I wasn't happy with my career but more painful was my girlfriend. I was with her for a few years and proposed a few times. I finally found out why she wouldn't marry me, she couldn't. She was having an affair the entire time and was already married! That killed me, I pushed her aside and there would be periods when I got so down I would literally call out of work and eat my pain away for a day straight. I would just eat"

John took his emotional eating and started doing something about it. He continued to make healthy eating decisions, and he more importantly started to measure his portions. I recommended he see a therapist about his issues. He again turned to pride and shame.

"I knew deep down inside of me that talking to someone else was going to be fruitless when it came to my ex. I was fat, I ate in an out of control manner, and I used her as nothing but an excuse. If I was going to stop emotional eating, I was going to have to fix the problem myself. I took James' recommendation of writing things down, and I wrote her and myself a letter. I called my mom as my dad had been gone for a few years and told her what my problem was. She felt horrible, but I needed her for help and not to feel bad.

I bought her a membership at the gym James trained at, and she started working out with her. James spoke with her and me about teaming up to conquer my emotional eating, and her boredom eating which it turns out is emotional eating as well. We meet for breakfast everyday and she calls me throughout my day to see how things are going. When I thought about Jenny, my ex, I would call mom instead of running to the fridge. It was rough for a few weeks, getting past not eating, but I did it.

I almost had a relapse, I did for a few days actually, when she showed me her divorce agreement. She wanted to be with me, and be my wife. It was an emotional overload, and I started eating. I did catch myself a few times and put my food away and called my mom. My mom made it a lot easier, and she even helped tell Jenny where she could go and how to get there in my mom's comedic fashion.

I still get sad, but I can tell you having someone to turn to and forcing myself to "feel better" was priceless. I demanded more respect and accountability from myself too, food needs to be seen as a "benefit" for health and fuel and not to use it as a crutch.

Write These Down

For the mirror, write this down and repeat it while looking at yourself. I was told by a training client that this over time invoked extreme respect for herself.

"You are NOT a loser or failure. In fact, I apologize for not respecting you more. This is my life and I AM gaining control of it, day by day."

These are other things you can write on your notes for the mirror:

"I did much better today than I did yesterday"

"I respect myself enough to keep pushing on"

"This is the start of a new approach toward success"

For the refrigerator or freezer use these:

"Did the alarm go off?"

"Did I earn a cheat yet?"

"Am I make a healthy choice? If not put it back
and scream
that you scored another win!"

"It's a snack, can I put off for a little bit
longer?"

"Do I need a ration now, or can I wait another
30 minutes?"

"Snack time, can I name 2 ways I went out of
my way to exercise?
No?! I will do that first and then come back."

For the credit card:

"Am I buying something at a fast food spot? I
should just tell them I forgot my credit card
and score a win"

"Is it time for a cheat? Put me back and cancel
the order."

"I really don't need to be used on a snack, buy
a fraction of a stock somewhere instead."

"I'm about to use this, but I really want a win
instead"

Write yourself a letter, an honest and heartfelt letter. I put mine under my mattress. It contains something that i am still dealing with emotionally, and have chose to keep it to myself. I did tell myself, using the loss as an excuse was no longer acceptable. I let myself know that there were going to be days when I knew I was going to quit my journey.

A Sample Journal

How many times did you beat the trigger this week? Did you see the trigger coming on? Did You stick to your plan? These are all things you should be taking account of.

Day	Food Consumed	Trigger	Did I Beat The Trigger? Why not?

What Can YOU Do?

As you've probably noticed, emotional eating can be caused by a seemingly unlimited number of triggers. I can't predict what you are suffering from, or if you even have an emotional eating problem. You, however can decide if you may. You can use an unlimited number of ways to combat your emotional eating using those above. Either Way, I would love to hear your story and successes, you may be published in our next edition!

Find us on Facebook at www.facebook.com/rrdunlimited
rrdunlimitedllc.info

Health Disclaimer

All material on this website is provided for your information only and may not be construed as medical advice or instruction. No action or inaction should be taken based solely on the contents of this information; instead, readers should consult appropriate health professionals on any matter relating to their health and well-being.

The information and opinions expressed here are believed to be accurate, based on the best judgment available to the authors, and readers who fail to consult with appropriate health authorities assume the risk of any injuries. In addition, the information and opinions expressed here do not necessarily reflect the views of every contributor to Emotional Eating. Wisdom Through Words acknowledges occasional differences in opinion and welcomes the exchange of different viewpoints. The publisher is not responsible for errors or omissions.

www.ingramcontent.com/pod-product-compliance
Lightning Source LLC
Chambersburg PA
CBHW070615290526
45790CB00002B/925